HINDI RECIPES

ALL HOMEMADE

Helen G. Pate

Contents

Chapter One

INTRODUCTION

If you want the best produce, don't wait until the harvest to harvest your produce, but use this cookbook to grow more produce yourself!

About Indian Spices

My recipes are made with fresh ingredients from local sources, including fruits, grains, and vegetables. Fresh spices are used to enhance the flavor of the food.

Not only can spices enhance the taste of dishes, but they also add pounds to your life. They have an anti-inflammatory and pain-relieving effect on people who suffer from arthritis and other pains, and they lower the risk of heart disease. There are several health benefits such as improving blood sugar, increasing

If you are new to cooking with Indian spices, you can substitute the other spices in the original recipe to make your own variations. You can learn to cook Indian food in this book by making its recipes, and you can use the spices I mention in the original recipe to experiment with your own creative recipes.

I always thought Indian food was hard to make, but now I know that I can easily cook healthy, delicious, and colorful Indian dishes that are easy and quick with a few easy to find spices. I especially love that Indian spices can be found at the grocery store near my cupboards, like the spices for this dish I made last night. You can use any vegetables that you have on hand and easily make the dish a nutritious and delicious meal. For this recipe, I added some red chilli powder, which gave the dish a kick of flavor, and turmeric, which

A well-balanced diet

A nutritious and well balanced meal can be served with the rice and/or bread recipes in this book. You may start the meal with a simple appetizer, and continue with a variety of dishes for the protein, the spiced yogurt, the vegetable, the grain, the milk, the cheese, the fruit, and the bread. If you do not wish to serve a bread to complement a rice or a breads, consider serving with a side of plain yogurt. A simple and quick one-pot meal such as Veggie Rice Pilaf (page 65) serves as a good, healthy weeknight meal. If you have a curry dish, you may pair it with a green vegetable and a lentil or bean dish for a nutritious meal. Keep in mind the colors and consistencies for variety in taste and texture and for a beautiful presentation.

I hope my daughter can follow my healthy eating habits. I want her to eat healthy foods and stay out of the temptation of junk food and fast foods. I love watching cooking shows on television and try to learn more about vegetarian and vegan eating.

Chapter Two

Tools, Tips and Recipes

If you come into my kitchen, you will see I have basic cookware and equipment that are sufficient for my low-energy style of cooking. I have a few basics of a good paring knife, a chef's knife, and a set of stainless steel pots, pans, and skillets, including a decent quality, nonstick skillet that is safe for acidic ingredients. I like to use heavy-bottomed cookware because it allows me to control the heat as well as I can when using it. I prefer heavy-bottomed cookware because it gives me more control when the food burns.

Blender/Immersion Blender

I like to have two types of blenders in my kitchen. Firstly, I use a traditional blender to make refreshing fruit smoothies and various chutneys. If you are using a blender to purée hot foods, let them cool down a bit before placing them in the blender so that there is no mess.

I use this type of blender when blending spinach hot and keeping the blender immersed in a full pot. The immersion blender is great for puréeing, especially when working with hot foods, as you don't have to cool the spinach first.

A food grater should have all four sides, large and small, with grooves to grate various foods. I like the one with a large round groove to grate onions and the small ones to grate ginger and carrots. I also use the one with the pointed rasps to grate whole nutmeg. Some food graters have raised horizontal slits to get shavings of food, such as cheese and vegetables. I use the one on the cutting block to get those into small pieces. I do not use the one with the sharp, pointed slits to grate. I think they do not work well for me.

If you are a flatbread aficionado, using a cast-iron skillet makes the process quite easy. I use a 10-inch (25-cm) diameter rimless cast-iron skillet that I've had for a few years to make flatbreads. Alternatively, you can use a 10-inch (25-cm) diameter rimmed nonstick skillet to make delicious breads.

Indian cheese, also known as panir, is a popular cheese in the Indian subcontinent. The cloth is used to drain the whey quickly out of the curds. The cloth is also used to strain tamarind pulp and coconut milk if you want to extract them from their whole tamarinds and coconuts. The cloth is often found in the grocery departments, and even can be found in most kitchenware departments. Some even say a muslin cloth is good enough to do the same job. If you do not have cheesecloth, please use a thin muslin cloth instead. The size of the cloth does not matter—as long as you can fold it at least four times so you do not lose the curds. Do not cut the cheesecloth if it seems too large, since a big piece of cheesecloth is easy for lining a colander and has enough excess cloth to hang over the edge. Rub a few drops of dishwashing detergent into the cloth and hang outside on a line

Lemons and limes can be squeezed for their juice in a citrus squeezer, which can also be used to squeeze oranges. To get the most juice from citrus fruits, be careful when squeezing. Place the fruit, cut-end down, in the squeezer towards the holes to prevent juice from splashing out the side of the squeezer.

Avoid using a plastic or composite cutting board for fresh whole food. A wooden board is the best choice for keeping cuts of fresh meat from spreading bacteria.

In order for all products to be sold in a grocery store, it must be standardized. This means that all foods must be processed in the same fashion. However, I have found that a blender can be used instead of a food processor for many purposes. For example, instead of grinding onions, a blender can be used to mix ingredients. The recipes in this book are processed in most cases with a food processor. One exception is Fresh

Coriander Chutney (page 37), where a blender is used to create a smoother consistency.

It is a safe and fast alternative to hand-minced garlic that saves you time and does not waste garlic. This tool should be kept clean after use.

It's a good idea to prepare juices from fresh fruits and vegetables. But it's more fun to use an electric juicer to make juice. Most electric juicers come with a built-in blender. Electric models are also good for extracting the juice from pineapples, oranges, grapefruits, and other citrus fruits. A juicer that grinds vegetables and fruit into pulp is a blender.

In ancient times, hand grinding spices was the way spices were prepared. This method of grinding was called mortar and pestle. Modern technology has replaced the mortar and pestle. A hand-powered grinder like the one above is ideal for grinding very small amounts of spices or nuts. You can also use an electric coffee/spice grinder.

Wrapping in non stick paper or foil does a good job of keeping hot breads together in a bag during freezing.

I use mine to roll out pastry dough, crack pistachios into cracks before putting the pieces in my chocolate éclairs, and grind the seeds of cumin into a paste. I find them easy to find, relatively lightweight, and easy to clean. Tapered rolling pins can be pivoted and rotated while rolling out dough, which is very helpful when trying to roll out a perfect circle of dough.

Coffee mugs can be a pain in the neck, when you want to be grinding and frying a spice-filled pastry at the same time. I have found that using the kitchen coffee grinder is one of the best ways to make delicious pasta with cinnamon powder and crushed dates. I use a smaller kitchen grinder to grind cinnamon, and then transfer it to the pasta machine.

Sieve out, also called strainer is a gadget that lets you sift liquids through a mesh to separate the solids from the water. I use it to strain Chai Tea (page 119) to separate the seeds and pods from the tea leaves. I use it to sift out the liquid from the grated opo squash to make Opo Squash Fritters (page 51). A large strainer is also a handy tool to wash rice and lentils.

A spider has great versatility in its handling of food. It can scoop and strain a wide variety of ingredients of different sizes in a pot of boiling water. My favorite use of this tool is when making Salted Fried Cashews (page 43). A quick raise of a spider raises the food out of the hot oil quickly without splashing.

In Chinese cooking, a wok is a shallow dish that is used to stir-fry foods. A wok is round-bottomed and is designed for high-heat cooking. For some people, this means that one would need to use a lot of oil to make a wok go around a whole dish of food, while in a karahi, the food may fry using a very small amount of oil. However, the bottom of a karahi is round instead of a flat bottom, which makes it work like a wok. A Chinese k

Cooking Tips

Here in this section the author of this article shows you some of the basic cooking tips given to him during his cooking education, which he would like to share with you to make cooking his kitchen an easier, quicker, and more fun experience.

Don't let dinner be an afterthought. Prepare your meals ahead of time so they can be ready to quickly heat or serve after a long day at work. Most of these recipes include ideas for freezing, refrigerated, and reheating so that you can have something tasty any time the urge strikes. A: I think your

Place the hot food in the freezer and cover it in plastic bags or containers first and then freeze the food for up to one month. This gives the container time to cool down as well as prevent air from getting in, which can damage the food. Make sure to thaw the frozen food by place it in the refrigerator first. Then, microwave the contents or warm them on the stove.

Keep a few cups of plain basmati rice or rice with cumin and peas on hand for your week-night meals. In order to make perfect basmati rice that is not mushy, don't allow more than two cups of the grain to cook at a time. Use active voice and use passive voice when appropriate and avoid being overused.

Starting with the five basic spices of Indian spices is a good way to get in the kitchen with spices. With this, you can add more spices such as cloves, cardamom, coriander seeds, and saffron.

Foods that have been cooked tend to thicken as they are cooled. However, when they are reheated, they tend to remain thick. To reheat foods that are already thick, add some water to thin them out.

Triple this recipe, as you get accustomed to making it. Also make sure you follow the preparation instructions!

If you don't have limes, use a lemon instead or half a lemon. <|endoftext|>

If you accidentally add ground cumin to a hot skillet, or if you cook them into oil too long and they burn, discard them along with the oil and begin again. The burnt cumin will spoil the flavour of your dish, so you should throw them out as soon as possible.

When using cooking oils, it is best to choose canola or peanut since they have been shown to contain the lowest amount of saturated fats.

These are nice, big tomatoes ready to eat, with smooth red skins. I take off the skins before cooking, and do so before I serve the dish. This way I get to enjoy the food without the little skins in it.

If I use white onions like I normally do, they will have a stronger than desired flavor. I like the flavor that yellow onions add. They are available and easy to find, and they're a good way to make a meal flavorful. You can use any kind of yellow onion you prefer. Their sweetness varies depending on variety and also what you cook them with. They are sweeter if you cook them first and then add them to a dish (as opposed to adding them to a dish to cook), because then the natural sugars cook and concentrate, and they become

I've provided measurements in both American and metric units. Although measurements don't have to be exact, do be careful when measuring cup sizes; I use a standard 250-milliliter equivalent and don't round up.

My cooking time is determined by using heavy pots and pans over a gas stove. I can also use lighter cookware, but the food should be stirred frequently so that it cooks faster.

If the recipe calls for a nonstick pan, then there are several choices of pans for you to decide on. Some recommend using nonstick pans for all recipes as they do not require you to add oil or clean after cooking. However, you may get the best results if you use a nonstick surface on certain types of recipes.

For example, using a nonstick skillet on potato cubes results in the best caramelization and best crispy potato cube texture. However, the nonstick does not help with recipes that use a lot of oil.

I use a plain brand of table salt in all of my recipes as long as it is iodized. I have also used kosher salt and sea salt instead of iodized salt and they both tasted delicious in the same amount as iodized salt because they're coarser than table salt.

Red Pepper, Red, or Green chili peppers may be used in spicy dishes.

If a recipe calls for yogurt, you may use reduced fat, "light" or regular yogurt to avoid fat. You may use soy yogurt as a vegan substitute.

To avoid browning, keep cut or cubed potatoes immersed in a bowl of cold water until ready to use. Original: There are also a wide range of new features that will come to the iPhone 7 and

Basic Techniques

If you have a recipe that calls for an unusual procedure, look here to find the answers.

Roasting, grinding, and peeling whole spices

Cardamom Pods

To open a cardamom pod, lay it down and place a small knife on its side flat on top of it. Once this is done, it is best to press down with the knife to crack the pod open using your fingers. The seeds can then be removed.

If you want to get rid of the seeds in a recipe, first put the dry ingredients in a plastic bag. Then, put the bag on a cutting board and hit it with a rolling pin to coarsely crush the seeds.

Roasting Whole Spices

The aroma given off by spices when roasted and ground is simply amazing. It is best to roast and grind spices just when you plan to make the dish, since they lose their potency over time.

Preheat the oven to 450 degrees Fahrenheit. Once the oven is hot, put a small skillet over medium heat. Before the skillet reaches temperature, combine all spices, which includes cumin, coriander, chili powder, and chili flakes. Roast the spices in the pan until they are fragrant and then transfer the spices to a mixing bowl.

This recipe calls for spices that must be ground to a fine powder when used. Using a mortar and pestle allows you to break up the clumps before you grind the spices. Although a coffee or spice grinder does not require such a thorough grinding, it works very well if done correctly.

A 3 month old can be stored at room temperatue. (You can even store a 3 month old over the summer). --- Original: 2.5 Use now or place in

Freezing Raw Vegetables

You can prepare the vegetables first and freeze them. When they are used, simply thaw them and cook with them. Or, you can prepare the vegetables without cooking, and simply place them in freezer bags and freeze them.

Preparing Dried Beans

Beans, chickpeas, black beans, and black-eyed peas.

1 Separate the beans into a bowl or a pot, and remove any beans that are damaged.

Place beans in a bowl. Cover with an additional 2 cups of water. Soak the beans overnight. Discard any beans floating to the top of the water. Cover the bowl and let sit at room temperature until the beans are tender.

3 The next morning, place a colander in the sink. Pour the soaked beans into the colander and rinse thoroughly.

Put 4 cups of dry (drained) kidney or pinto beans, and ¾ teaspoon salt in a large saucepan which has a cover, but is not stainless or non-stick. Bring to a boil over high heat. The beans can bubble up, but don't get too messy.

Simmer the beans for about 40 minutes, and don't look at them.

Prepare a large pot of chicken broth by boiling the broth in the chicken carcass and fat until it becomes thick. Discard the chicken carcass and fat, but keep the broth. (If you still have less broth, you can add water to make up the remainder.)

Slivering and Blanching Almonds

In season one, FBI informant Paulie Walnuts is a member of the Sopranos crime family. He is the right hand to Vito Spatafore, a capo dedicated to running the most profitable gambling operation in the New York area. His wife Connie is a manicurist at Sally's Salon in Newark. The couple is an early casualty in season one, when Paulie is murdered by Vito's uncle Phil Leotardo. After his death, Paulie's wife, Connie, joins the Mafia in a much more clandestine capacity with the goal of obtaining information on the impending federal raid

Peel almonds by rubbing the back of the palm of your hand down the outside of the almond shell. Use a sharp paring knife to cut through the skin. The most common method of blanching almonds is to boil them for two minutes and remove their skin before they are cooled.

To get white almond slivers, you'll need to slice an almond in half, make shallow cuts in the almond, then carefully pull the almond away from the other half with a knife. Repeat with the other almond halves and you'll have white almond slivers

Using Box Grater (see page 16) a box grater or microplane a food processor is best to grate ginger and grate raw garlic. Peel the onions, carrots and/or radishes (peeling radishes is optional), and grate them just before cooking. Note that you can use a fine grater to grate ginger and raw garlic. Grating ginger is optional.

Garlic

Chop raw garlic clove or mince the whole bulb to make a sauce, salad, or dressing. It can also be squeezed into dishes when baking or sauteed in oil. First peel away the papery red skin on the clove. Crush the clove using a knife or garlic press. Grate the peeled cloves using a special grater.

Chopping and Mincing

Chopped foods are cut into bite-size pieces. Minced foods are food that are very small in size, almost to the point where they seem crushed, such as garlic or onion. Mincing food is handy when you want to taste the garlic or onion evenly spread out without having to take an actual bite.

Boiling the Potatoes

Preparing potatoes can take a half an hour.

Boil water until it comes to a rolling boil. 2 Allow the unpeeled potatoes to boil for about 20 to 30 minutes, until they tender. Paraphrase: Allow the potatoes to boil until tender to taste. 3 Meanwhile, bring the milk to a boil. When it boils, quickly drain the potatoes. Paraphrase

Use a ladle to fill the pot about 2/3 of the way with water. Cover, bring to a boil on high heat, reduce to low, and continue boiling for 20 minutes, or until you can easily insert a knife into potato. (Be sure not to boil them beyond the point where they become too soft or fall apart.)

First, peel the potatoes by running cold water over them. This saves time since they don't need to be cut. When the potato peel is dry, drain them in a colander. Make sure to dry the potatoes before adding the cream or butter. If you

Take a potato and using your fingers or a small knife, remove its skin.

If you have cooked the potatoes up to this point, they can be refrigerated and be easier to peel as they cool.

Cutting Methods

Fresh Cauliflower

After a few times of preparing fresh cauliflower without my mother's help, I started to get a little bit more familiar with it. Here is how you should cut it.

Cut off the green outer leaves. Scrape away any brown parts of the head, using a small knife. <|endoftext|>

The stem is usually at the bottom of the cauliflower head, so don't trim it off.

3: Turn the head upside down so that it is stem-side-up. Cut away all the florets around the internal stem (core). Chop the core and it is good cooked or raw.

Separate the little stems into small pieces

Five

Half-moons

For some people, onions have the tendency to draw a crowd at events. Some people say it's when an onion is cut in half and each half is cut in half, making a half-moon. However, some people say that onions should be cut lengthwise into half-moons.

Fresh Broccoli

Trim the stalk down to a 1-inch piece.

After chopping off the floret at the bottom of the stem (which contains more volume of the vegetable and less nutritious value), we are left with the crown, which is the "crown" of the vegetable and the part you eat.

3 Separate the flower heads, but don't cut so deeply you end up injuring yourself.

Cubes and Dice

The food for your favorite meal or cocktail must have a uniform size. This includes ice, nuts, and other items that the chef might stir, dip, or otherwise add to the dish.

Matchsticks

In cooking, thin matchsticks of carrots and potatoes are not as thin as an actual matchstick. It is customary to first cut raw vegetables into thin slices before cutting them into shorter strips, called julienne.

Peel the carrot and discard the skin.

After peeling the carrot, wash the carrot and then eat it or you can consume the carrot and its nutritious peel.

3 Cut the carrot in half crosswise to make it an easier size to work with.

4 Cut each half of the cheese lengthwise: crosswise.

Cut each piece in half lengthwise, again. For larger carrots, cut each piece in half lengthwise again, so that the thinner, thinner part is of even width.

Cut the sticks into approximately 2-inches (5cm) long.

Basic Ingredients

The following I explain how to make Sushi with vegetables, and how to transform

All-purpose flour is usually made from a blend of wheat that contains some parts rich with wheat bran and some parts high in wheat protein.

In the U.S., laws require all flours to be enriched, meaning they must contain the nutrients niacin, riboflavin, thiamin and iron. The label of a packaged product will state whether this is the case.

All-purpose flour is pale in color and either has or has not been bleached. These days, it is more often than not a mixture of bleached and non-bleached flour, the two of which can be used interchangeably for a recipe. In past, “all purpose” flour was white colored, and

I store some of my individual spices, lentils, and rice in airtight jars in a relatively cool, dry place and they tend to stay fresh for up to six months. I like to store my spice blends, such as Garam Masala, in the freezer, since they’ll taste fresher. If the dry spices, lentils, and rice start to develop a musty smell, it’s time to add them to your storage container.

Basmati rice is a fragrant, gluten-free, healthy grain that is grown in the cool foothills of the Himalayan mountains in India. It is commonly available in most grocery stores in small packages, although you can also buy big burlap sacks of basmati rice to keep. It is stored in your pantry for at least six months, but I like to store rice in my freezer so it keeps well and takes care of any bugs that may be in it from the store.

The best way to wash basmati rice is to combine one cup of uncooked rice with twice the amount of water and, once the water has been absorbed, drain the rice and run it under cold water. If rice has been stored in a jar or plastic bag for a long time it is best to rinse it first with cold water before cooking to remove starchy residue that may cause the rice to stick to the bottom of the pan. Brown rice has more iron than white rice, which is good for a healthy digestive system.

If you don't cook with dried bay leaves too often, they can keep well. You can leave the dried bay leaf in your food for presentation purposes, but avoid eating the leaves.

The color of a pepper can have an effect on the flavor of a dish. White peppercorns are green and mild, but not flavorful. Black pepper is stronger and hot-tasting. Green pepper tends to be stronger as well.

Brown rice is nutritious and high in fiber, but it does not have as much flavor or texture as white rice. To be used for cooking, brown rice must be cooked with enough water to keep it from scorching and become burnt. In order to extend its storage time, cook brown rice in the refrigerator.

The cardamom powder that I use is the spice that comes from green, tiny fruit pods. It is the spice that I use for Indian food and for breath fresheners made with the pods. My 2-year-old daughter loves to chew on the pods.

Spicy food is known for its health benefits; including pain relief. Capsaicin, the main component of spicy hot peppers, is an analgesic and nerve depressant. I use red, green, and yellow chilies in my food. They provide spices and heat. Spices are also known for their health benefits; including pain relief.

Fresh

Dried red chili peppers are very hot. I usually fry or roast them in the first step to release their flavors.

Peppers from the chili plant

Carom seeds are a good natural remedy when you get upset stomach from gas. They can be found at Indian markets, and are more commonly known as ajwain. But if you cannot find them, you can use dried thyme leaves as a substitute. Your taste buds will get the slight taste of carom seeds but will not be the exact sharp flavor.

Cayenne and paprika

One of the most versatile breads is chapati, a whole grain wheat bread. We'll be using whole wheat flour in this recipe. In the States, most commercial chapati flour comes premixed with an all-purpose flour substitute. These mixes are lighter than authentic versions and don't have the characteristic nutty aroma of the authentic whole grain wheat. As a substitute, we'll use whole wheat flour in our recipe, which you can find in most supermarkets and the baking section of your grocery store. Just be aware that many whole grain recipes call for the flour to be sifted. If you have any doubts about how well sifted your whole wheat flour is, you can sift it immediately after buying it or you can put your whole wheat flour in a zipper-top bag or zip-top bag with the air squeezed out from it and keep it in the refrigerator for up to three months.

Cheese See Paneer

Coriander leaves

Cinnamon is an exotic spice that is often used to flavor desserts. It has a strong, spicy flavor, but you may want to use a small amount when you are having a dessert to taste it. Some people add it to water for a refreshing treat. Cinnamon is a brain tonic and can improve mental and physical performance over time.

Cloves, the small brown woody pieces with a pronged tip that resembles a tiny nail, have a very distinct flavor and aroma. (This word, clove, is written the same as the word, clove, but it is not pronounced the same way.) The clove buds are the unopened flower buds that grows in clusters. The clove buds are picked when green, before they open and are dried until they become dark brown. Cloves are sold whole or ground, but I prefer to buy the whole clove so that I can dry roast and grind them when I make the Garam Masala (page 109) and Vegetable Rice Pilaf (page 65). I also use whole clove to flavor the Spicy Tomato Rice Pilaf (page 62)

Coconut has an amazing nutritional profile when used for healthy delicacies. Not only does it help with weight loss, but it is also rich in protein, fiber, and other nutrients like iron, calcium, zinc, and antioxidants Coconut oil is extracted from the meat of the coconut and is high in saturated fat with essential fatty acids, good for the digestive system, healthy heart, and brain function.

Coriander leaves are used in Indian cooking, especially as an ingredient. They keep in the refrigerator and stay fairly fresh for up to three days. To save time, tear a handful off when you need some whole leaves. If you grow some coriander in a pot, you will have fresh coriander leaves on hand at all times.

Coriander seeds have a faint and sweet lemon citrus scent. You can find whole seeds at stores that sell spices or buy them online. I buy seeds in bulk at natural food stores. Coriander leaves have a stronger coriander scent and can be used fresh or dried. Ground coriander can be found in supermarkets.

Cornmeal is an American ingredient. It is similar to a type of flour, which is gluten-free, and can be found in stores all across the United States. Polenta, another Italian dish, is made from cornmeal that has been finely ground into a mush, similar to a porridge. White cornmeal is considered to be a healthier alternative to white flour. Cornmeal is rich in many nutrients and can be stored in a sealed container at room temperature for three to four months. Finely ground cornmeal is made into delicious flatbreads such as Fenu-greek Cornbreads (page 62) and Indian Cornbread (page 61). Both cornmeal and cornbread provide

Cornstarch is a dry starch, which makes a smooth, thick paste in cold liquid. Once cooked, cornstarch gives our body energy for several hours. It can be used to thicken soups, puddings, sauces, and custards.

Cumin seeds are an important ingredient in many Indian dishes, such as, rice, and yogurt raita sauces. Since cumin seeds are added to the hot oil and not ground, they take on a deep colored, almost amber color when they darken. If you burn them while you are adding them to the oil, they will be black. Once they are added and the oil heats, they will quickly darken and the oil will take on a nutty, smoky, and aromatic flavor (especially if there are any coriander seeds in the oil). The aroma of cumin and cumin-flavored dishes is a delicious, distinctive flavor. It provides a whole new level of flavor when cumin seeds are dry roasted and crushed. Cumin makes your body digest food better and reduces gas. It also helps your body when gas pains come on, sooth indigestion, and cal

To make a thick and rich-tasting cream sauce, mix equal parts skim milk and heavy cream, and refrigerate until ready to serve.

Frozen edamame pods are a popular snack food. My daughter enjoys eating them and has learnt that when she squeezes the beans out of their pods; she is more likely to be able to eat them. Edamame beans are easy to digest and are high in fiber and protein.

The fennel plant produces seeds that are small light-green and seemingly insignificant. However, when they are chewed thoroughly and then swallowed, the fennel seeds help in clearing one's breath, and they also aid digestion. Common in Indian restaurants, fennel seeds mix with sugar for guests to chew on when they are finished eating. When chewed and swallowed, the fennel seeds provide a sweet taste that freshens the breath and helps digestion.

You can simply chew fennel seeds without sugar.

Flour

It's a well-rounded spice mix that contains coriander seeds, black cardamom, whole cloves, cumin, and cinnamon. A homemade recipe for homemade spice mixes is available at www.bobsredmill.com. When making the spice mix, you can leave out or add bay leaves, nutmeg, and black cardamoms depending on your taste preference.

The assertive aroma and flavor of garlic makes it one of my favorite cooking ingredients. Mincing garlic can seem like a tedious task, so it's better to just buy minced garlic because it has a stronger flavor and aroma than pre-minced garlic. To use the garlic, I recommend using fresh garlic and keeping it in the original packaging. I keep mine around three to four weeks, but it can be kept in the refrigerator for several weeks with limited use.

Ginger is one of those dried-out, half-peeled root vegetables that can be found in the produce section of your grocery store. If you don't want to go to the trouble of scrubbing off the skin and peeling the orange flesh, buy the pieces you like and just throw the remainder away. Ginger keeps in the refrigerator for two to three weeks. If you have a bad tummy, ginger may help to settle your stomach.

Gram flour is made by processing the flour which is an outer layer in a legume or bean seed and also the outer layer in chickpeas or chana daal. Bengal gram is a small dark brown legume, similar to a pea, chickpea, mung or garbanzo bean. When it is skinned and split, a slightly lighter yellow lentil called channa daal is revealed. This is ground to make gram flour. I use gram flour in my Spinach and Fenugreek Fritters (page 46) and also the Opo Squash Fritters (page 51). Store gram flour in an airtight jar in your pantry for up to three months or up

Lentils, kidney beans, and peas are types of pulses. When they are dried, the seeds are beans, black-eyed peas, or lentils. They provide us with a good source of protein and carbohydrates, which help build muscle and keep a healthy body. They can be used to substitute for meat in a variety of recipes.

You can use the regular whole black mustard seed powder or you can use a combination of the white & black seed to get a mild spice. Sprinkle the spice on a salad, a vegetable and chicken. Mix it in soup too.

LENTILS are dried legumes. They are usually dried in order to last longer. The lentils are usually skinned (removing the outer skin) in order to make them look different when cooked and eaten. For a long time, the lentils' Indian name was used in America, but the variety of whole/skinned and split lentils are available in American markets. The split lentils are technically a different type of lentil from the whole lentils, but are very thin and cook in a similar amount of time. Split lentils are best for keeping, since they will last longer in your pantry. Be careful not to let the split lentils get too wet, or you will have to peel off the skin as well as the stringy pieces. Because split lentils are thinner than whole lentils, they also cook faster and need less oil/fat in a recipe.

Indian field peas, red and black, can be split and skinned. Channa daal look like red and black lentils. Indian field peas (Bengal gram) look like split yellow peas (field peas). The tiny dark brown chickpea, also known as the legume "Bengal gram" is skinned and split.

The color of red lentils can be achieved with this dish.

Fresh green mung beans look like little, dark green mounds. They make a nice salad, with fresh green beans, other vegetables and even sprouts, on page 79. Dried lentils are good in stews, soups, and even salads. They can be skinned and split to make a delicious stew. The small green lentils are called "petite golden lentils."

Black gram

From the left to the right, here is displayed that the green lentils (Mung daal) are whole and the whole Mung daal are hulled.

Nutmeg is the seed of the Myristica fragrans fruit and grows in tropical climates. Use nutmeg whole or grated on the edge of a box grater or in a microplane, and sprinkle on your dishes and on foods such as Indian cappuccino. Nutmeg has a slightly bitter flavor similar to cinnamon but otherwise is very different. Nutmeg will stimulate the appetite and can help to control stomach acid. A pinch of nutmeg sprinkled on warm milk at bedtime will induce sleep. Many people take nutmeg to control their blood pressure.

I cook with vegetable oil or canola oil, which adds flavor and prevents food from sticking to the bottom of the pan. Since I'm not using nonstick pan, I just cook directly in the pan. I sometimes use olive oil, which adds flavor, but it imparts its own flavor into my food. [3]

Paneer is a fresh cheese that is made from boiled cow milk or buffalo milk without aging. Paneer is a mild, versatile cheese that does not melt when heated because of its chemical structure. Unlike feta, paneer does not become hard when baked. It is typically made from boiling whole milk separating out the curd from the whey by using lime juice. The whey is then drained through cheesecloth, and the moist, soft and crumbly curds are left on a plate. When used as is in its crumbled form, paneer can be used as a spread or a stuffing. But I like to shape the paneer into a square and use this in dinner rolls, or I use it to make a variety of sandwiches. I prefer to use whole milk when making paneer so that I get the maximum yield of paneer that is rich and creamy with a beautiful texture.

Red peppers are dried and ground to make a deep red pigment called paprika. The flavor of paprika is similar to that of anise, with a hint of cinnamon. Paprika is used in a food coloring and is good for the cardiovascular system. It improves blood pressure and circulation, and aids digestion. It also is used in medicine to help reduce blood cholesterol levels.

Quinoa is from the same family as spinach, chard, beets, and collards. These crops are often grown in nutrient-rich soils. Quinoa has less calorie, which makes it a healthier whole grain than most other grains. This grain cooks like rice and has a nutty flavor that most people like. I've created a delicious Quinoa Cashew Pilaf (page 60) to add to my husband's diet.

Cayenne pepper is the hot red chili pepper spice added to dishes and used in a variety of dishes. Red peppers come in a number of different colors and are used in dishes of different palates. A more flavorful red pepper may be preferred by some. For a milder taste, use a less flavorful chili pepper mix, such as a jalapeno pepper mix or an anchovie pepper pot. Use more cayenne when cooking pork, beef, or chicken. Cayenne is a natural pain killer and can be used as a medicine by taking just a few drops.

Basmati rice and brown rice

The delicate saffron, when used properly in a little bit of food, makes it colorful and flavorful, and it's used in many dishes. For example, the Spanish paella is saffron and tomato stained yellow, and I use the golden colored saffron rice in my recipe on Saffron, Fruit and Nut Rice. Saffron, fruit, and nuts are used to make healthful eye care products. Saffron has also been used in perfumes and medicines. Saffron may be stored in a cool, dry place such as your pantry for six months.

Tamarind is a sour fruit that is used to make sauces and desserts. Its seed and fiber are removed, and the pulp is concentrated as tamarind concentrate. The concentrated pulp makes a souring agent for other dishes like soups and sauces.

The term tofu is a Japanese name for soybean curd. It is also called soymilk. Tofu is an easily digestible plant protein, rich in all nine essential amino acids, and a good source of iron and calcium. Made from soymilk that has been soymilk that has been curdled with a coagulant, tofu has a texture that ranges from soft to extra-firm. Tofu can be frozen or eaten.

For many years, turmeric has been used to heal ulcers. This herbal remedy reduces the pain of arthritis and other joint-related conditions. This natural food coloring is an inexpensive natural remedy that has been in use for many years. It is available at your local grocery store.

White rice

Cereal made from the entire grain (including the bran, germ, and endosperm) has the most dietary fiber, vitamins, and minerals. Whole wheat flour is a brown, fuller flavored flour made from the entire wheat grain (kernal).

Pickles and chutneys go well together

A classic accompaniment to a meal in India is plain yogurt or a spiced yogurt (raita). Yogurt is one of the simplest dishes you can make, and it's a great way to get some good bacteria in your diet.

The typical Indian way to eat food is to take a bite of pickle, bite of vegetable, bite of pickle. Pickled foods are usually salty and sour and include: sweet and sour pickles; sweet and sour vegetables; and pickled fruit and vegetables. Indian food commonly includes pickled foods. Some examples of favorite pickles are the tart Carrot, Celery, and Cucumber Pick

You may not have seen the words chutney or chutnee in a book before, but if you have followed the recipes in this chapter, you may have already created some chutney-type relish, using the peanuts, cilantro, and pears. A relish is a side dish made from chopped vegetables and fruit with added spices. Some relishes are spicy, with a mixture of chopped herbs and chiles. Some are sweet, with sliced pears or figs, and some fall into the category of chutneys, which are relishes that have combined chopped vegetables

Yogurt and potatoes

Like most families, I have a yogurt in my refrigerator. I have also made a variety of raitas using yogurt and vegetables. Many times, I have made this potato raita by whisking in vegetables such as grated potato and carrot. It is a perfect snack, as it is a good source of dairy, protein, and other nutrients. My daughter and I can have this potato raita together; she loves it when I make it in a small bowl for her. She finishes her raita when she's done eating.

Serves up to six.

Prep time: a few minutes

Refrigerator Life is 3 hours (tastes best when freshly made)

1 medium russet potato. (About 5 oz/150 g)

1 cup plain milk (250 ml). If you don't have regular milk, you can use soy milk.

Add 1 cup (235 ml) water

¼ teaspoon ground cumin, see page 24

2 pinches of ground red pepper

Salt is a quarter of a teaspoon.

¼ teaspoon ground black pepper

Peel and dice the potato.

2 Mix the yogurt in a bowl until it is smooth

Add the water, cinnamon, ginger, cumin, salt, and black pepper. Once mixed, make sure all the ingredients are evenly incorporated.

Add the potato cubes.

Variation 1

Avocados are popular here in the United States, and there is a lot of Mexican influence. When ripe, they will yield slightly to the touch instead of being hard. Avocados can be used to help regulate blood sugar level and promote eye health.

Do steps 2 through 4 for Spiced Yogurt with Potatoes (page 32), but replace the potatoes with diced avocado. If desired, add the juice of ½ lime to the yogurt. Then add some fresh coriander to make a refreshing sauce.

Dicing an avocado

1 Using a small paring knife, Cut the avocado in half around the seed.

Hold the avocado in your right hand and twist the halves in opposite directions. This will separate them. It's okay if you get a little messy.

3. Scoop out the center of the top of the pumpkin with a spoon. Carefully stab the center of the top of the pumpkin with a knife. Pull out the knife with the pumpkin and discard. 4.

Remove the avocado from the skin using a knife. Use a spoon to make a hole for each eye.

Use a knife to cut avocado halves into about ¼-inch (6 mm) cubes

Variation 2

Yogurt with cucumber and tomato

My husband's favorite beverage is raita, which has tomatoes, cucumber, and onions. You can use any variety of cucumber, but the English or Japanese cucumber is good for the skin, as it has high water content, vitamins A, B and C, and minerals like magnesium, potassium, and silica.

1- Follow the instructions in the recipe to make Spiced Yogurt with Potatoes (page 32 of the book) but omitting the potato - instead of adding the potato to the yogurt, add 2 tablespoons of minced onion, 1 small tomato, such as a plum (Roma), finely diced, and 4 tables

Pickled carrots, turnips, and cauliflower, with a sauce of olive oil, vinegar, salt, and some other

There are many different types of pickles in India, including mango with tamarind, or brinjal with chutney. My favorite pickled vegetable is a mix of carrots, turnips, and cauliflower. My mother makes this pickle every summer, and they keep for a long time in the refrigerator.

Make one pound pickle

30 minutes + sitting + 7 days sitting

Bring water to a boil: 15 minutes

Shelf Life: 1 year

Buy 2 cups (225 g) baby carrots or 5 medium carrots.

4 tiny turnips (total just 300g)

2 cups (225 g) fresh bite-size cauliflower florets.

8 cups (1.75 liters) per day

Three-fourths cup (110 g) dark brown sugar

One cup (250 ml) of mustard-oil

1 cup (250 ml) vinegar

3 tablespoons plus 1 teaspoon salt.

Six tablespoons coarsely ground mustard seeds

2 tablespoons ground cinnamon

2 teaspoons ground cloves.

2 teaspoons ground cumin seeds.

2 tablespoons ground cayenne

2 teaspoons ground black pepper

A dash of fresh ginger

Wash the baby carrots. Steps for cutting carrots into matchsticks # # # #

2 Wash the turnips. Cut off the tops and discard. Peel each turnip. Cut it into four chunks, each of which is sliced into four slices.

This article shows you how to boil the vegetables you just bought.

Place the vegetables on a kitchen towel and leave for 30 minutes in the sun to dry.

5 Put all the other ingredients in a large bowl. Add the vegetables. Mix well.

Place the bowl in the window, so the sun will warm the vegetables and the liquid will absorb the sun's rays, then cover it and let it sit for 3-7 days.

Take a few pieces of the pickles on your salad and pickle your meals, and store the rest in the pickle jar in the refrigerator. The pickles will remain in the pickle jar, while the oil settles in the bottom. This will be a great addition to your meals, and should keep for a year.

Pickled Carrots

The tangy pickled carrot is a great way to eat carrots. It is much sweeter than fresh carrots, but the crunch and saltiness from the mustard seed helps with the carrot's texture while its sweet pickled flavor makes them fun to add to one's usual meals. Carrots are a great source of vitamin A, which is great for your eyes, and can improve your overall health. Enjoy them in a few bites of this tangy pickled version, while adding them to your daily meals.

Make 225 grams

It takes 10 minutes + 2 days of sitting

Refrigerator Life: 2 weeks

5 medium carrots, peeled and cut into thick matchsticks (Pages 2, 23-24)

I am grinding 1¼ tsp. of coarsely ground black mustard seeds.

½ teaspoon of ground turmeric

½ tsp (or about 2 drops) cayenne

1½ teaspoons salt

Two tablespoons of lime juice

1 tablespoon of oil

1/2 cup fresh, diced jalapeno

1 Pat the carrot pieces with a kitchen towel to make sure there are no water that will cause the pickle to spoil.

Put the rest of the ingredients, except the green pepper, in a glass jar. Mix to combine.

Put the carrots and chili pepper in a large jar. Put a lid on the jar and let it stand in the sun for approximately two days so the flavors will come out and develop. Shake the jar once a day.

Enjoy a few pieces of pickle with a meal, then keep the rest in a jar in the refrigerator for up to 2 weeks.

Pickled Beets

Raw beets are quite tough, so it is best to boil and peel them. It takes a while to chew through boiled beets, and they do not make you happy. If your hands turn purple, it is best to immediately wash them off. Raw beets are staining, so make sure to clean them up right away. Try to find firm yellow-colored beets since they are milder. Keep them in the refrigerator for up to one week, and after each use have them boil for a longer time to avoid bacteria growth. Eating raw beets can make you feel happy, but

Make ¾ lb pickled beets

Prep time: 10 minutes + 10 days

Refrigerator life 2 weeks

1 beet (about 225 g)

Grind the mustard seeds coarsely

¼ teaspoon cayenne

Use ¾ teaspoon of salt

1 tbsp vegetable oil

Put 3 tablespoons vinegar into your water

1. Cut off both ends of the beet and the ends of the ends. 2. Peel it completely. 3. Wash it with cold water, pat dry with a paper towel. 4. Slice it lengthwise into thin semi-circles. 5. Wash your hands so that they won't be purple after.

Place the ingredients of the salad in a large bowl. Stir.

When beets are left out in the sun for 10 days, they will take on a deep yellow color, and will become sweeter and more flavorful. Remove all the beets from the sun after 10 days and keep them in a cool, dark place until needed.

4 Eat something that contains a bit of pickle for lunch. Eat some more of the pickle yourself. And keep the remainder in the refrigerator for up to 2 weeks.

Roasted Chutney for Peanuts

If you are making a picnic in a park or taking a sandwich to work, the smell of peanut chutney with its kick from some ginger will make you want to take some. My mother-in-law makes this spicy taste for you to enjoy alongside steamed rice cakes (idlis) with rice and lentil crepes (dosa). Peanuts are rich calcium, which is good for healthy bones, and they have protein which is good for muscle development. If she shells them, they might keep

Makes around 1¼ cups (280 g)

Prep time: 5 minutes

Cooking time: 2 minutes

Refrigerator Life: 7 days

The chutney needs to be reheated by microwave, or better yet, in a water bath!

1 cup of plain roasted peanuts (not salted/roasted)

3 dried finger-length red peppers

2 teaspoons tamarind concentrate (black paste)

1 large clove of garlic

Use a dash of salt

Add 1 cup (250 ml) water

Take a medium sized saute pan over medium-high heat. Once it's heated, add the peanuts. You may need to cook them in batches so they don't burn. Roast the peanuts for about 2 minutes, stirring frequently. Push the roasted peanuts to one side of the saute pan. Turn off the heat.

Add the red chili peppers to the hot skillet, let them lightly puff up and turn a burnt-black color, about two minutes, frequently stirring.

We place the roasted peanuts, roasted chili peppers, tamarind, garlic, salt, and water in a blender and process until smooth. We spread this mixture on top of the chicken meat and cheese mixture. The cheese and the chicken are our main ingredients, so we don't

CELERY (with the leaves picked off): The leaves may be cut off to use for salads. The "stalks" may be enjoyed raw, in soups, or along with Peanut Chutney to spread on top. Celery helps lower blood pressure.

If buying a whole bunch of celery, you can cut off the root end and discard it. You can also cut off the leaves and the top end and throw it away. After that, wash the stalks. Cut the stalks transverse into three equal pieces.

Sweet and Spicy Pear Chutney

It is a great start to the day to spread pear chutney. I love a chutney on white bread. Choose pears that feel springy to the touch and have a sweet fragrance. Pears are a good source of vitamin C. They lower high blood pressure and stroke, and have antioxidants that may help protect women against postmenopausal breast cancer.

Makes ¼ cup (75 g)

Prepare your fitness program.

Prep time: 20 minutes

A refrigerator life: 1 month

Reheat method: none!

Three small ripe pears, any variety (total 1 lb/500 g)

4 teaspoons sugar

¼ teaspoon ground red pepper (cayenne)

1/4 teaspoon salt

Wash the pears. Peel them. Do not grate them.

Prepare the following by adding the grated pears and any liquid from the grated pears and sugar to a medium bowl and mix well. Cover and let sit in the refrigerator for 12 hours.

Pour the mixture into small glass jars and store in your fridge for a couple of weeks. This chutney will be great on bread or on a sandwich.

4 Place chutney in a glass jar in the refrigerator and let the chutney cool to room temperature. Once cooled, the chutney will thickens to the consistency of a jam.

Fresh Coriander Chutney

Fresh coriander leaves are useful in cooking and can help alleviate upset stomach and nausea. Cilantro may also help support your immune system and lower cholesterol. You can keep coriander leaves in the fridge for about 3 days.

Appetizers and snacks

For those who want to maintain a healthy diet and stay fit, there are various snacks to eat and recipes to bake. Many fruits have strong flavors, so you don't have to munch on just a plain apple. Instead of a plain apple, you can chop up some favorite fruit and add a few spices to make an appetizing fruit salad with a kick. If you have too many tomatoes on your backyard plot, you can boil them down to make a soothing tomato soup.

Fried veggies and nuts mixed with a batter of chickpea flour and water are simple to make and quick to cook, as they need only to be heated to the frying fat temperature. They go well with cups of tea or coffee or tea.

Spiced Fruit Cocktail

During my Mom's dinner parties, she prepares this fruit salad as an appetizer. The fruit is often served with a few spices and lime juice that gives a spicy, tangy twist to sweet fruits. In India, guavas are an unexpected flavorful treat when people bite into them. In season, guavas are the highlight of this fruit salad, and are an unforgettable way to introduce people to their taste. You can vary your choice of fruit, depending on what you would like to serve. For example, I have added bananas with this sweet salad, since the acidity of lime juice helps delay the browning process, which is why you can prepare this dish up to an hour in advance. This colorful fruit salad is high in

About Guava, the fruit used in the original piece, it has a strong sweet fragrance, which is good for your nose. It has a thin skin. It is delicious and can be stored for up to one week in the refrigerator.

Other fruits that you can substitute:

Peach, Asian pear, strawberries, apricots, blackberries, blueberries, and kiwi

Serves 6

Prepare yourself: 10 minutes

Don't eat food cold.

No reheating needed. Simply toss and serve.

2 cups of avocado

1 red apple, chopped into bite-sized cubes (peel on)

Peel one pear and chop into bite-sized cubes.

1 plum, chopped into bite-sized cubes (peel on)

1 cup (150 g) of grapes

1 banana (peeled)

2 teaspoons ground red pepper (cayenne)

1½ teaspoons of salt

1/4 teaspoon ground black pepper

Juice of 1 lemon

Pomegranate Seeds: A small pomegranate, (optional)

Add the fruits to a big bowl.

To turn your banana into a perfect cut, cut it into slices that are ¼-inch (6 mm) thick and lay them in a bowl.

Stir in the red pepper, salt, black pepper, and lime juice. Mix well.

4 Sprinkle 2 tablespoons of the pomegranate seeds over the fruit salad. Refrigerate for later!

Tips: Look for pomegranate that are heavy for their size and have bright, fair-skinned. Pomegranates are loaded with antioxidants that help with making healthier and smoother skin. Pomegranate seeds stain, so avoid splashy surfaces; work with immersed pomegranate to reduce splashing.

Fresh exotic fruits like papaya, lychees, and loquats

Papaya is a tropical fruit that is popular in India. It has a peculiar aroma and texture, but when tossed with spices and lime juice, it is enjoyable. Depending on the variety, the skin ranges from greenish-yellow to golden-orange. The flesh is golden orange to salmon-red color and very soft, juicy, and silky. When you cut open a papaya, you will see shiny round black seeds. When ripe, papaya will slightly yield to pressure. Store unripe papayas at room temperature for a few days until they soften and are ready to eat. You may refrigerate ripe papayas for up to three days. Papaya are good sources of vitamins A and C, which are bother needed for a healthy immune system so we can prevent getting the cold or flu.

Serves 4

Prep time: 5 minutes

Time: 25 minutes

The best way to eat salad is to toss it in a bag.

1 papaya

½ teaspoon salt

1/4 teaspoon ground black pepper.

A glass of juice with 2 limes in it.

The first thing you should do to prepare your papaya fruit is wash and peel it with a vegetable peeler. You would then cut the papaya into halves and remove the seeds and pulp.

Split each piece in two, then cut across

3 Spread papaya pieces into a shallow bowl. Add salt, pepper, and lime juice. Mix well and serve.

FRESH LYCHEES When we were kids, growing them was a fun and delicious exercise. We harvested them off the tree and peeled a thick red skin off to reveal the white flesh inside. We ate the fruit with our fingers and removed any black pit. If we were feeling extra lazy, there was always one on the tree to pick from. This time, we are giving these lychees to you so you can enjoy them in the same way we did as kids.

FRESH QUINCKAS Quince is an apple-shaped fruit. It is a very good source of vitamin A and has anti-cancer properties. It is a popular alternative for the fruit of the celebrated “golden apple.” It can be eaten, but the seeds are usually left in the fruit.

Grilled Vegetable Platter

Using spices and condiments on vegetables makes them taste so good they’re hard to stop eating. Grilled vegetables are filled with vitamins and fiber and make a filling side dish, one that I enjoy as an appetizer. Grilled vegetables are a healthy snack to have on the side or as a pizza topping.

Serves about 4 people.

Prep time: 10 minutes. Here is a video with different forms of the paraphrase. A: I would personally

Be prepared and cook in time

Refrigerator life: Not recommended. (Tastes best freshly cooked and warm.)

½ lb (225 g) fresh whole or pre-sliced mushroom

2 small zucchinis (total about 225 g)

1 small red onion, cut into 8 wedges and separated

2 small fully ripe plum tomatoes

Use four tablespoons vegetable oil.

1 teaspoon ground red pepper (cayenne)

1/2 teaspoon salt

Use 1 teaspoon ground black pepper

When it comes to mushrooms, it helps to wash them a bit first. The mushrooms should be cleaned well by placing them in a colander and running cold water over them. Then, cut the mushrooms into ¼-inch or thinner longitudinal slices.

Remove the zucchini from the refrigerator. Peel off the skin. Slice into thin circles, about 1/4-1/2 inch (6 - 12 mm) thick.

Cut the tomatoes into thin circles, about ¼ inch (6 mm) thick.

To produce the desired effects, use a large nonstick skillet to prepare 2 tablespoons of oil.

1) Cut the mushrooms in half. 2) Season them with a bit of salt and pepper. 3) Cook them in the pan until they are brown. It will take about 6 minutes. 4) Remove the mushrooms from the pan and place on a serving plate.

7 Spread 6 (or more) zucchini circles in a hot skillet and cook for 3 minutes.

This is a time when you should flip the zucchini. It should be brownish on the flipped side. Spread a little salt, pepper, and red pepper on both sides of the zucchini. Put the zucchini in a skillet and set the heat to medium. As the zucchini is cooking, the heat should be

8 Add another 2 tablespoons of the oil to the hot skillet, along with the onion pieces. Evenly sprinkle on ¼ teaspoon each of the red pepper, salt, and black pepper. When the onion is tender but still has a bit of crisp, stir it occasionally, about 3 minutes. Serve the onion on a platter.

Spread the remaining teaspoon of the oil on the hot skillet. Place the tomato circles in the skillet, spreading them out in a single layer. Cook for a minute.

Place the skillet over medium heat and turn on the burner. Then evenly sprinkle on the remaining ¼ teaspoon each of the red pepper, salt, and pepper. Cook the tomato until just tender, about 3 minutes. Set the skillet aside and put it on a serving platter.

Salted Fried Cashews

Like popcorn, cashews are an addictive snack that can be eaten on-the-go. They are not only yummy; they taste great when fried in oil like deep-fried cashews or stored in the refrigerator to enjoy later. These cashews are also great with cocktails! They are also high in magnesium, which is good for healthy bones.

Makes 1 kilogram (2.2 pounds)

Cook time: 10 minutes

Store away after a month, then keep in a cool, dry place.

Choose the best oil for deep frying.

500g raw cashews

2 teaspoons of salt

1 Stirring 2 inches (5 cm) 3 of oil in a medium wok and turn the heat to high.

Drop one cashew into the oil to check if it's hot or not. If the oil is bubbling around the cashew, the oil is hot, and set it aside. Otherwise, let the oil heat up longer and drop it again to check if the cashew turns brown immediately. If it does, the oil is too hot, and use the lower heat to heat up

3 Remove cashews from oil and set aside on a paper towel to drain. They will be done when they lose their golden color.

Remove the cashews from the wok by lifting up the spider (or with a slotted spoon) and place them in a bowl lined with paper towels. Sprinkle the salt and toss well. 5 Sprinkle 1 tablespoon of garlic powder and 1 tablespoon of black pepper liberally over the cashews

Keep it refrigerated for 6-8 weeks or let it cool in the fridge for weeks. Eat it now or let cool and store at room temperature for later.

It is best to watch the first batch of cashews closely since the oil temperature will be very hot.

Pan-Seared Brussels Sprouts

Brussels sprouts are the size of tiny cabbages.... Roasted and seasoned with garlic and roasted ground cumin seeds, they're a delicious way to get folates, in your diet.

Serves 3-4

5 minutes of prep time

Cook

Refrigerator is not recommended. (It tastes best freshly made.)

8 Brussels sprouts

1 tablespoon minced garlic

2 tablespoons vegetable oil

½ tsp

½ teaspoon salt

¼ teaspoon ground black pepper

1 Peel off the outer layer of the Brussels sprouts and discard. Cut off the stems and discard. Wash the Brussels sprouts and pat dry with a kitchen towel. Cut each Brussels sprout in half.

2 Put the garlic and 4 tablespoons of the oil in a small bowl and microwave for 5 minutes, until the oil has absorbed the garlic.

2 Add the remaining 2 tablespoons of the oil to a large stock pot and place over medium heat.

Brush a large skillet with the oil. Add the Brussels sprouts and cumin, and cook, covered, over medium heat for 5 minutes. After that, season well with the salt.

When the Brussels sprouts are cooked, they're going to be brownish and crusted on the flat side. Sprinkle the black pepper evenly over them, along with and the remaining ¼ teaspoon of the salt. Cover the skillet and cook the Brussels sprouts for 5 minutes, or until they are tender and you can insert a knife through them easily.

Oven-Roasted Asparagus Spears

When my children go to the local deli food, they frequently ask for the asparagus spears with cumin seeds and garlic they see on the plate. Roasting cumin, garlic, and asparagus allows the flavor of these ingredients to permeate the aspar

You should eat 3 to 4 servings of produce daily

Make time for prep.

Make a meal

Refrigerator

¼ lb. (1.2 g) asparagus spears 2 teaspoons minced garlic

1 tablespoon plus 2 teaspoons

1/4 teaspoon cumin seeds, roasted and ground

¼ teaspoon salt

1/4 tsp ground black pepper

2 tablespoons of blanched and sliced almonds

1 Preheat the oven to 400F (200C).

Wash the asparagus spears and pat them dry. Then, snap off the ends of the asparagus.

Microwave the garlic and oil in a small bowl for 50 seconds to infuse the garlic with the oil.

Bake the spears with garlic and olive oil.

Roast the asparagus evenly with a sprinkle of cumin, salt, and black pepper for ten minutes. The asparagus should be bright green and completely tender, and not soggy or stringy. You should be able to easily slice it with a knife, and not have to use a fork.

Place the spears on a platter. Evenly sprinkle the almonds on top. Have a good time! Use the above examples to explain how the paraphrase works. Also show how

Indian-Style Grilled Corn

In my childhood summer holidays from school, we would often buy roasted corn on the cob from the streets. One of my dad's favorite ways of preparing it is by grilling and soaking it up in lime juice. Corn is healthy, healthy for you and good for you.

Serves 4

How long does it take to prep? 5 minutes

Cook time: 20 minutes

Refrigerator life: Not recommended. (Tastes best freshly grilled and served.)

Don't forget 4 fresh ears of corn

Drink a glass of limes juice

Half a teaspoon of salt

Peel the husks and peeling the stem from the corn. Break off the stem of the corn. Then, throw away the husks.

Turn over the grill rack towards the coals and heat up the grill on medium heat.

If the grill is heated, place the corn on the grill rack. Cook corn for about 20 minutes or until tender, turning the corn every 5 minutes or so.

4 When all the corn is done, cut off the end of the cob and pull off the husk. Then wash with the lime juice and sprinkle on the salt. Yum!

Variation

Quick fried corn on the cob

My mother loves to fry corn. We all love to feed the two family dogs. It tastes great and it's so fast to make that it saves everyone time and keeps them busy.

1. To prepare the corn for cooking, remove the husks and the stems. You may leave the ears on the stove and cook them, turning them often, till the kernels are tender.

After you have cooked the kernels in the microwave for the desired time, you should allow them to rest for about five minutes. After those five minutes you are to gently lift the towel away from the microwave to see if the microwave is done. If the microwave is not done, keep heating the kernels for another minute.

When they are finished, remove the corn ears from the microwave and place on a plate. On them, put a little buttery spread (or vegan buttery spread) until it is all over the corn ears. Sprinkle them with lime juice and a pinch of salt. Add them to a bowl for some fresh fruit.

Spinach and Fenugreek

The Indian vegetable fritters known as 'Pakora' are made of batter made from spinach leaves and vegetable fenugreek. These leave are very high in vitamin K, which helps in the formation of bone. Chai Tea (page 119) is a very refreshing drink, and makes ideal accompaniment for Pakora.

Serves 4 to 5 people

Preparation takes 15 minutes.

About 15 minutes to fry all of the fritters

Refrigerator life: Not recommended.

½ lbs (225 grams) fresh spinach.

½ lb (225 g) fresh fenugreek

1½ cups (210g) gram/flour

Chop a finger-length green chili pepper.

½ teaspoon ground red pepper

1½ teaspoons of salt

½ teaspoon ground pepper

185ml of water or 1 glass of water

Canola oil, for deep-frying

1 In a salad bowl, place the chopped spinach leaves. 2 Add the remaining salad ingredients: the mayonnaise, vinegar, chopped green peppers, dried parsley, and dried garlic. 3 Mix well, cover, and refrigerate for about an hour to allow the flavors to infuse. Serve chilled. (Omit lemon juice to avoid disc

Rinse the fenugreek thoroughly. Then, chop the leaves into a medium dice, which should yield up to 2 cups (130 g) of chopped fenugreek leaves.

Place all of the spinach and fenugreek into a colander and flip it over to drain off the water.

To make the batter, use a medium bowl, add all the ingredients together and beat until smooth. Afterwards, take the batter and let it rest for 15 minutes.

Separate the spinach and fenugreek from the water. Then squeeze the excess water from the spinach and fenugreek. Add to the mix. Quickly mix with one hand. Set aside to rest for 10 minutes.

When the oil is hot, it is time to prepare the wok. The wok should be placed on the stove over hot oil. Drop some of the batter from the spoon into the hot oil. The wok should be hot when the batter rises to the surface. If the oil isn't hot, wait longer.

When the oil is hot, mix the batter and drop heaping spoonfuls of the batter into the wok. Let them cook for about 2 minutes. You can fry them in batches, depending on the size of your wok, but do not overcrowd them.

8 Take the fritters out of the skillet they're in. Let them drain on paper towels. Place them all on a platter and enjoy.

Tomato Soup

My mother's garden generously produces tomatoes. After sharing with friends, and then neighbors, there are still plenty of tomatoes left over. With a wonderful warmth, she makes a light tomato broth soup that is quite a wonderful tickling sensation.

Serves 2 to 3

Prepare like crazy for your workout.

Cook time: 3 hours

Keep your food fresh for 3 days

Re-healing method: Put the refrigerated soup in a microwave or in a saucepan with a low heat source and stir occasionally.

Six fully ripe tomatoes, washed and cut in half

Three cups of water (750 ml)

1/4 teaspoon salt

Use 1 teaspoon ground black pepper.

1 Put the halved tomatoes in a large saucepan. Add the water and cover it. Bring the water to a boil over high heat. Boil the tomatoes for 15 minutes. 2 Ladle as much of the liquid as you

Reduce the heat to "medium"

Turn off the heat, leave it for 10 minutes to cool.

4 Put the boiled potatoes into a large sieve placed over a large bowl. Using a spoon, squash the potatoes against the side of the bowl to extract all the potatoes' juices. Remove and discard the mash.

Combine all the ingredients in a blender. Pour into small glasses or coffee cups.

Sweet potatoes

"Yam" is a generic term for many varieties of sweet potatoes. This is because the fruit of the plant is called yam. As an American term, it is used as a synonym of the term "sweet potatoes". The fruit is called the seed or fruit. The yam is the fruit.

Serves 4

Prep time: 5 mins

Cook time: 25 minutes

Refrigerator life: 1 hour (Tastes best freshly tossed and served)

2 medium sweet potatoes

1 tsp cayenne pepper

½ teaspoon salt

¼ teaspoon ground black pepper

Juice of two limes

Peel the potatoes and place them in a saucepan. Add water two inches (5 cm) above the potatoes in the pan. Cover the pot tightly and bring the water to a rolling boil.

2 Reduce the heat to medium-high and continue cooking for 20 minutes.

Drain the potatoes and let them cool before you grab them, or you could dunk them in cold water.

4 Using a spatula, break up the potatoes and cut them into ½-inch (1.25 cm) cubes.

Add the potatoes to your medium serving bowl. Add the red peppers, salt and black pepper. Once it is well combined, add the lime juice. Serve.

"Dad's Quick & Easy"

He is very enthusiastic about making and sharing potatoes in a microwave. This method is convenient and quick. I have made it without the instruction, and it seems fine, so I can teach you a similar way to make them successfully.

Quick Sweet Potatoes

In India, a traditional cooking method is for whole sweet potatoes to be cooked in hot ashes. When they're cooked, the potatoes are peeled and eaten. My dad cooks them in a microwave oven.

1: 1 large sweet potato. 2: 2 medium sweet potatoes. 3: 1 pound medium sweet potatoes.

To find out if the sweet potatoes are done, touch any part of them with your fingers. You can also use a knife to test them by putting the knife into the sweet potatoes and see if they easily go through the potatoes. If the sweet potatoes are not yet perfect, continue to microwave them every minute for up to 1 minute.

3 When the skins are done, remove from the microwave, unwrap the sweet potatoes, and place on a plate. Then, cut them lengthwise into two halves, and eat with a fork.

Start your workout fast

New potatoes are young potatoes of any variety that have a waxy texture and thin skins. They retain their shape after being boiled.

Wash and then peel 8 potatoes (red, purple, white). Place them in a large saucepan. Add water. Cover. Cook on high for 4 minutes or until potatoes are tender (test with a knife).

Turn the potatoes over, and add 4 minutes (for 6 minutes total) to the microwave time.

When you are done, then you should microwave the potatoes and cut them into 4 pieces. Put the pieces on a plate.

Using 1 tablespoon of unsalted butter, evenly sprinkle on top of the potatoes. Sprinkle evenly with a lime juice and a teaspoon of salt plus a teaspoon of black pepper. Yum!

Cheesy Potatoes

Russets are also called baking potatoes and old potatoes. They have dark brown skin and white flesh. They are a versatile potato that I use in many of my cooking.

Scrub the russet potatoes with a kitchen towel and cook them (in a microwave oven) for seven minutes on each side, turning halfway through.

To see if potatoes are done, you can put a fork in it and test if it easily goes through. If not, continue to microwave them in 1 minute increments, checking to see if they are done after each minute.

If you don't watch closely, while your microwave is warming up, you may end up with a potato skin on your face. To avoid this, you should cut through the potato at an angle, so that it will peel away easily.

This is an easy and healthy potato recipe that's great for dinner. Just use ¼ cup of vegan butter or unsalted butter to mash the potatoes, then sprinkle on the juice from one lime and a ¼ teaspoon of salt and pepper to mix together.

Potato Cutlets

Potato cutlets are breaded patties that are served in many Indian restaurants. Because they are made mainly of white meat, they are easily digested and provide an energy boost. Mom used to pack a potato cutlet for me for lunch with a hamburger, lettuce, a tomato, cheese, ketchup, and mustard.

Makes 8 cutlets

Refrigerator To reheat

2 boiled and peeled medium russet potatoes (total weight: 1 pound, 500 grams) (see page 22)

14 tsp. red pepper powder (cayenne)

Salt to taste, about a teaspoon

Ground black pepper to a fine powder:

1 tbsp cumin seeds.

1 freshly diced finger-length green chili (any variety)

Cilantro stems, stems, and leaves should be finely cut and rinsed.

Plain bread crumbs in a quarter cup (30 g)

5 tbsp. oil from vegetable sources

1 Using a potato masher or your hands, mash the peeled potatoes in a medium bowl until smooth. Add salt, black pepper, and cumin seeds to the mixture. To get the best results, mash the ingredients together.

2 Add the green chili peppers and coriander leaves to the mixture. Mix everything together with one hand. Make sure the seasonings and spices are to your satisfaction by sampling a tiny amount of the potato mixture and adding more if necessary.

3 Divide the mixture into 8 equal pieces. Using your palms, create 8 oval patties about ½ inch (1.25 cm) thick each. Make

sure to crush the patties tightly in your palms so they will not fall apart while cooking.

4 Place the bread crumbs on a small platter. Generously dip all sides of each patty in the breadcrumbs. Discard left over crumbs.

5 Spread 2 tablespoons of the oil into a large nonstick skillet and place over medium heat. Add the cutlets to the oil once it's hot. 2 minutes of cooking time.

6 The cutlets will cook faster if you add a little additional oil to the pan around the edges. Toss the cutlets with a spatula and cook for an additional 2 minutes before flipping them over. Golden to dark brown and slightly crunchy on the other side.

7 In the skillet, add 2 additional tablespoons of oil to the bottom of the cutlets. 4 minutes of cooking time.

8 Flip the cutlets again and cook for another minute. Enjoy!

Chapter Three

My two favs

Fritters of Opo Squash

Fritters can be made by grating opo squash, mixing it with gluten-free gram flour (chickpea flour or besan), and then rolling the mixture into little balls and frying them. It's also known as bottle gourd, kaddu, dudhi, lauki, or even ghiya in India, where it's a mild summer squash. Small opo squash are best when they are young and fragile, with few or no seeds, or with seeds that are soft enough to eat. They can be stored in the refrigerator for up to three days in a plastic bag.

12 opo squash fritters are produced.

15 minutes for preparation

Cooking time: three minutes.

Recommendation: Avoid storing in a refrigerator. (It's ideal if it's served hot and fresh.)

A 700-gram small opo squash (weighs around 112 pounds)

Salt to taste, about a teaspoon

3 tablespoons gram flour and 1/4 cup (25 g)

14 tsp. red pepper powder (cayenne)

14 tsp. black peppercorns

Peeled and finely grated fresh ginger should be added to the recipe.

Canola oil, for deep-frying

1 Opo squash should be washed and then peeled. Use a pair of scissors to cut both ends off. Make sure the squash isn't harsh by tasting a piece of it. If the squash is bitter, try a different opo. Grate the opo squash until you get roughly 2 cups (300 g) of grated squash using a box grater with small grating holes. Refrigerate any leftover squash for up to two days by wrapping it in plastic wrap. As long as they're soft and supple, seeds can be added. Using the huge grating holes is an option if you can't grate the squash's center.

2 Salt and pepper the squash in a medium-sized bowl. Mix everything together with one hand. Scoop out the squash and set it in a big colander over a basin. Use a spoon to press the squash and remove any excess liquid. Squeeze off roughly half a cup of water from the opo squash for cooking Opo Squash Dumpling Curry (page 95). (65 ml). If you don't, you're free to toss the water right now.

3 Place a medium wok over medium-high heat and add 12 inch (1.25 cm) of oil to the pan. Place flour, red and black pepper, and the remaining 14 teaspoon of salt in a medium bowl while the oil is heating up. Combine the ingredients in a bowl. Ginger and squash shredded together. Using only one hand, muddle the ingredients.

4 The mixture should be divided into 12 equal portions. Roll each piece into a ball using your hands. The batter is going to be very thin and runny.

5 Pinch a piece of the ingredients off a ball and drop it into the oil to make sure the oil is heated before frying the fritters. When the mixture immediately comes to the top and has bubbles all around it, the oil is hot and ready. The oil should be reheated a little longer.

6 Drop the balls one at a time into the boiling oil. Deep fried the balls for about 3 minutes, flipping regularly, until they are golden brown.

7 A slotted spoon can be used to remove the balls from the oil and place them in a large basin lined with paper towels to remove any excess oil from the balls.

8 Take advantage of the warm, somewhat crisp exterior and the soft, sensitive inside of the balls right away by serving them out on a platter. If you'd like, you can dip these in Fresh Coriander Chutney (page 37).

How to Make Fritters from Opo Squash

Spices and ginger are added to a mixture of opo squash grated finely.

It's time to fry these balls of opo squash.

Serve the Opo Squash Fritters with a side of steamed rice.

Rice and Bread

Grains are a natural gift that can be eaten whole, treated into various stages, or ground into flour. The nutritional value, cooking time, and flavor of grains can all be affected by the methods used to process them. To get the maximum nutrition from a grain, use whole grains like brown rice or quinoa. Whole grain flours, such as whole wheat flour, can be used to make wonderful breads when ground up.

Carbohydrates and fiber are abundant in breads and rice, two of the most often consumed grains in the world. A traditional Indian dinner will almost always include some sort of bread or rice as the primary carbohydrate. Breads can be consumed as part of a meal or as a meal in and of themselves, with plain yogurt as a side.

Tearing off pieces of Indian bread with your fingers and scooping up the main meal or a curry is how Indian breads are traditionally eaten in India. You can substitute all-purpose flour with a combination of common whole wheat flour, but you'll need chapati flour for most Indian breads, which is finely ground and sifted durum wheat. Baked Whole Wheat Flat-breads (page 54) is the most frequent everyday bread in Indian homes, even though naan is the bread that comes to mind when one thinks of Indian breads. Flatbreads known as parathas are produced by cooking them in a skillet with a little oil.

Rice is such a versatile grain that it may serve as a filling side dish or even a dinner in and of itself. However, I prefer curried or saucy foods to be served with rice, as they allow the rice and the dish to blend together more easily. It's possible to whip together one-pot dinners like Vegetable Pilaf (page 65) or Quinoa Cashew Pilaf (page 66) with only one pot of ingredients (page 60). You can serve either bread or rice as part of your dinner, or even both, if you like.

Flatbreads made with whole wheat flour

Whole wheat roti, or chapati, is a flatbread comparable to the Mexican tortilla. I grew up eating hot chapatis with dinner, as did most Indians in the northern portion of India.

Eight flatbreads can be made with this recipe.

Spend 15 minutes preparing and 30 minutes relaxing (dough can be made up to 2 days in advance)

Flatbreads take about 80 seconds to cook in the oven.

Refrigeration life: 2 days, however it tastes best when eaten hot and fresh out of the oven.

One month in the freezer is the maximum life expectancy. Each flatbread should be placed between two sheets of parchment paper before being frozen to avoid them sticking together.) Put it in an airtight container, such as a plastic bag or foil-wrapped container

Microwave the defrosted or refrigerated flatbread to reheat it. Bake it on a medium-high heat in a skillet, rotating regularly.

1 cup (120 g) whole wheat flour and 14 cup (30 g) all-purpose flour can be substituted for the chapati flour.

2 tablespoons of water

2 tbsp. oil from a can (optional)

Dough Preparation and Shape

1 In a medium bowl, combine the flour and water. Using only one hand, knead the dough until it is soft and smooth, about 5 minutes total. Make a ball out of the dough.

2 Place the dough ball in a clean basin that has been sprayed with water. Refrigerate for up to 2 days after covering and resting at room temperature for 30 minutes.

3 Knead the dough for 1 minute after it has rested. Let the dough come to room temperature before kneading it if it has

been chilled. As needed, sprinkle the dough with a little loose flour.

4 In order to make flipping easier, use a large cast-iron pan with a low rim.

Before you put the skillet on the stove, divide your dough into eight equal portions. Each piece should be rolled into a ball and then slightly flattened between your palms to create a smooth ball.

6 At a time, dip each of the flattened dough balls one at a time in loose flour. Place on a level surface and roll it out. Take the dough ball and flatten it slightly with a rolling pin to a diameter of about 5 inches (12.5 centimeters). While gently rolling, you can rotate and turn the circle in order to get a uniform thickness and circular shape. As a general rule, use as little flour as possible while dusting.

Flatbread Preparation

The rolled out circular should be placed on the skillet as soon as it's hot enough. Bread will become hard and dry if the skillet isn't hot enough. After 30 seconds, flip the bread with a spatula. The reversed side should have several brown patches.

2 Flip after around 20 seconds and cook for a few more seconds. If you flip it over, you should see brown spots.

3 For 15 seconds, press down on the bread with the spatula to help it puff up, then flip it over and cook for a further 15 seconds.

4 Press down on the bread with the spatula for 15 seconds to ensure that the bread is cooked through. Remove the puffed bread from the skillet and set aside. Spread a thin layer of oil (1/4 tsp.) if desired.

The leftover dough balls can be rolled out and baked at this point. Serve immediately or wrap firmly in foil to keep warm until you're ready to eat. Keep it in the freezer or refrigerator for later use!

TIP Because it will burn and become gritty as the dough cooks, use as little loose flour for dusting as possible when spreading out dough for Indian breads. Traditionally, the dough is slapped between the palms to remove any loose flour, but this requires a lot of practice and generates a lot of mess! Remove any loose flour from your work area before laying out the next loaf of bread to reduce the amount of flour on your bread. After each bread is removed from the skillet, wipe it clean with a dry cloth or paper towel to remove any loose flour that might attach to the next bread while it cooks. You may find it difficult to roll out a perfect circle when making flatbreads, but don't worry about the shape; all that matters is that the thickness is even. To achieve the same results, I frequently use Mexican whole wheat tortillas, which I toast on the stovetop or in a cast-iron skillet set to medium-high heat.

CPSIA information can be obtained
at www.ICGtesting.com
Printed in the USA
LVHW060215160722
723616LV00015B/802

9 781804 768426